GW00976526

THE ULTIMATE PLANT BASED DIET COOKBOOK
2021

Kick-start your journey with fast and mouth-watering recipes for beginners. Lose Weight and Heal your body in a few steps.

Ursa Males

TABLE OF CONTENTS

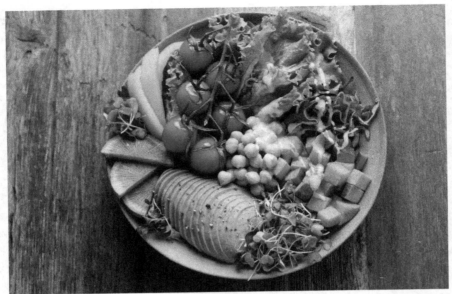

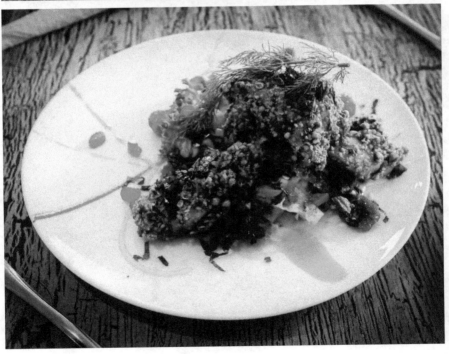

BREAKFAST

1. <u>Oatmeal and Carrot Cake</u>

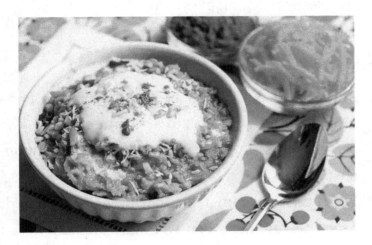

Preparation Time: 5 minutes

Cooking Time: 10 minutes

Servings: 2

Ingredients:

- 1 cup of water
- ½ teaspoon of cinnamon
- 1 cup of rolled oats
- Salt
- ¼ cup of raisins
- ½ cup of shredded carrots
- 1 cup of non-dairy milk

- ¼ teaspoon of allspice
- ½ teaspoon of vanilla extract
- Toppings:
- ¼ cup of chopped walnuts
- 2 tablespoons of maple syrup
- 2 tablespoons of shredded coconut

Directions:

1. Put a small pot on low heat and bring the non-dairy milk, oats, and water to a simmer. Now, add the carrots, vanilla extract, raisins, salt, cinnamon, and allspice.
2. You need to simmer all the ingredients, but do not forget to stir them. You will know that they are ready when the liquid is fully absorbed into all the ingredients (in about 7-10 minutes).
3. Transfer the thickened dish to bowls. You can top them with coconut or walnuts. This nutritious bowl will allow you to kickstart your day.

Nutrition: Calories: 210 Fat: 11g Carbs: 42g Protein: 4g

2. <u>Almond Butter Banana Overnight Oats</u>

Preparation Time: 5 minutes

Cooking Time: 10 minutes

Servings: 2

Ingredients:

- ½ cup rolled oats
- 1 cup almond milk
- 1 tablespoon chia seeds
- ¼ teaspoon vanilla extract
- ½ teaspoon ground cinnamon
- 1 tablespoon honey or maple syrup
- 1 banana, sliced
- 2 tablespoons natural almond butter

Directions:

1. Put the oats, milk, chia seeds, vanilla, cinnamon, and honey in a large bowl. Stir to combine, then divide half of the mixture between two bowls.
2. Top with the banana and peanut butter, then add the remaining mixture. Cover then pop into the fridge overnight. Serve and enjoy.

Nutrition: Calories: 227 Fat: 11g Carbs: 35g Protein: 7g

3. <u>Peach & Chia Seed Breakfast Parfait</u>

Preparation Time: 5 minutes

Cooking Time: 10 minutes

Servings: 4

Ingredients:

- ¼ cup chia seeds
- 1 tablespoon pure maple syrup
- 1 cup of coconut milk
- 1 teaspoon ground cinnamon
- 3 medium peaches, diced small
- 2/3 cup granola

Directions:

1. Find a small bowl and add the chia seeds, maple syrup, and coconut milk. Stir well, then cover and pop into the fridge for at least one hour.
2. Find another bowl, add the peaches and sprinkle with the cinnamon. Pop to one side. When it's time to serve, take two glasses, and pour the chia mixture between the two.
3. Sprinkle the granola over the top, keeping a tiny amount to one side to use to decorate later.

4. Top with the peaches and the reserved granola and serve.

Nutrition: Calories: 260 Fat: 13g Carbs: 22g Protein: 6g

4. <u>Avocado Toast with White Beans</u>

Preparation Time: 5 minutes

Cooking Time: 6 minutes

Servings: 4

Ingredients:

- ½ cup canned white beans, drained and rinsed
- 2 teaspoons tahini paste
- 2 teaspoons lemon juice
- ½ teaspoon salt
- ½ avocado, peeled and pit removed
- 4 slices whole-grain bread, toasted
- ½ cup grape tomatoes, cut in half

Directions:

1. Grab a small bowl and add the beans, tahini, ½ the lemon juice, and ½ the salt. Mash with a fork. Take another bowl and add the avocado and the remaining lemon juice and salt. Mash together.
2. Place your toast onto a flat surface and add the mashed beans, spreading well.

3. Top with the avocado and the sliced tomatoes, then serve and enjoy.

Nutrition: Calories: 140 Fat: 5g Carbs: 13g Protein: 5g

5. __Oatmeal & Peanut Butter Breakfast Bar__

Preparation Time: 10 minutes

Cooking Time: 0 minutes

Servings: 8

Ingredients:

- 1 ½ cups date, pit removed
- ½ cup peanut butter
- ½ cup old-fashioned rolled oats

Directions:

1. Grease a baking tin and pop to one side. Grab your food processor, add the dates, and whizz until chopped.
2. Add the peanut butter and the oats and pulse. Scoop into the baking tin, then pop into the fridge or freezer until set. Serve and enjoy.

Nutrition: Calories: 232 Fat: 9g Carbs: 32g Protein: 8g

6. <u>Chocolate Chip Banana Pancake</u>

Preparation Time: 15 minutes

Cooking Time: 3 minutes

Servings: 6

Ingredients:

- 1 large ripe banana, mashed
- 2 tablespoons coconut sugar
- 3 tablespoons coconut oil, melted
- 1 cup of coconut milk
- 1 ½ cups whole wheat flour
- 1 teaspoon baking soda
- ½ cup vegan chocolate chips
- Olive oil, for frying

Directions:

1. Grab a large bowl and add the banana, sugar, oil, and milk. Stir well. Add the flour and baking soda and stir again until combined.
2. Add the chocolate chips and fold through, then pop to one side. Put a skillet over medium heat and add a drop of oil.
3. Pour ¼ of the batter into the pan and move the pan to cover. Cook for 3 minutes, then flip and cook on the

other side. Repeat with the remaining pancakes, then serve and enjoy.

Nutrition: Calories: 105 Fat: 13g Carbs: 23g Protein: 5g

7. <u>Blueberry Smoothie Bowl</u>

Preparation time: 5 minutes

Cooking time: 0 minutes

Servings: 2

Ingredients:

- 1 tbsp. ground flaxseed
- 1 medium banana
- 4 ice cubes
- 1 cup blueberries
- ¾ cup unsweetened almond milk
- 1 tbsp. maple syrup
- ¼ cup nuts chopped

Directions

1. Blend all ingredients in a high-speed blender. Garnish with chopped nuts and mint leaves. Serve and enjoy!

Nutrition: Calories: 335 Carbs: 61g Fat: 5g Protein: 10g

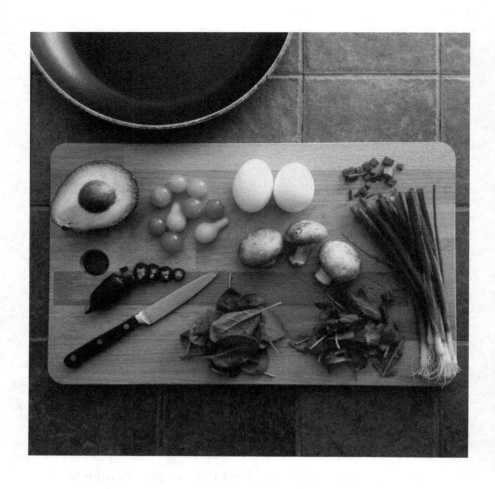

LUNCH

8. Spinach and Broccoli Soup

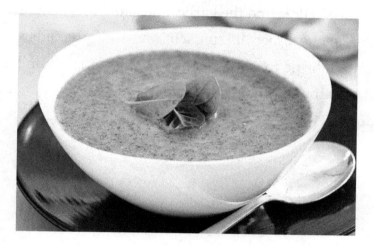

Preparation time: 10 minutes

Cooking time: 20 minutes

Servings: 4

Ingredients:

- 3 shallots, chopped
- 1 tablespoon olive oil
- 2 garlic cloves, minced
- ½ pound broccoli florets
- ½ pound baby spinach
- Salt and black pepper to the taste
- 4 cups veggie stock

- 1 teaspoon turmeric powder
- 1 tablespoon lime juice

Directions:

1. Heat-up a pot with the oil over medium-high heat, add the shallots and the garlic, and sauté for 5 minutes.
2. Add the broccoli, spinach, and the other ingredients, toss, bring to a simmer and cook over medium heat for 15 minutes. Ladle into soup bowls and serve.

Nutrition: Calories 150 Fat 3g Carbs 3g Protein 7g

9. **Coconut Zucchini Cream**

Preparation time: 10 minutes

Cooking time: 25 minutes

Servings: 4

Ingredients:

- 1-pound zucchinis, roughly chopped
- 2 tablespoons avocado oil
- 4 scallions, chopped
- Salt and black pepper to the taste
- 6 cups veggie stock
- 1 teaspoon basil, dried
- 1 teaspoon cumin, ground
- 3 garlic cloves, minced
- ¾ cup coconut cream
- 1 tablespoon dill, chopped

Directions:

1. Heat-up a pot with the oil over medium-high heat, add the scallions and the garlic, and sauté for 5 minutes.
2. Add the rest of the ingredients, stir, bring to a simmer and cook over medium heat for 20 minutes more. Blend the soup using an immersion blender, ladle into bowls and serve.

Nutrition: Calories 160 Fat 4g Carbs 4g Protein 8g

10.   Zucchini and Cauliflower Soup

Preparation time: 10 minutes

Cooking time: 25 minutes

Servings: 4

Ingredients:

- 4 scallions, chopped
- 1 teaspoon ginger, grated
- 2 tablespoons olive oil
- 1-pound zucchinis, sliced
- 2 cups cauliflower florets
- Salt and black pepper to the taste
- 6 cups veggie stock
- 1 garlic clove, minced
- 1 tablespoon lemon juice
- 1 cup coconut cream

Directions:

1. Heat-up a pot with the oil over medium heat and add the scallions, ginger, garlic, and sauté for 5 minutes.
2. Add the rest of the ingredients, bring to a simmer and cook over medium heat for 20 minutes.   Blend everything using an immersion blender, ladle into soup bowls and serve.

Nutrition: Calories 154 Fat 12g Carbs 5g Protein 4g

11.   Chard Soup

Preparation time: 10 minutes

Cooking time: 25 minutes

Servings: 4

Ingredients:

- 1-pound Swiss chard, chopped
- ½ cup shallots, chopped
- 1 tablespoon avocado oil
- 1 teaspoon cumin, ground
- 1 teaspoon rosemary, dried
- 1 teaspoon basil, dried
- 2 garlic cloves, minced
- Salt and black pepper to the taste
- 6 cups vegetable stock
- 1 tablespoon tomato passata
- 1 tablespoon cilantro, chopped

Directions:

1. Heat-up a pan with the oil over medium heat, add the shallots and the garlic, and sauté for 5 minutes.
2. Add the swiss chard and the other ingredients, toss, bring to a simmer and cook over medium heat for 20 minutes more. Divide the soup into bowls and serve.

Nutrition: Calories 232 Fat 23g Carbs 4g Protein 3g

12. <u>Avocado, Pine Nuts, and Chard Salad</u>

Preparation time: 5 minutes

Cooking time: 15 minutes

Servings: 4

Ingredients:

- 1-pound swiss chard, roughly chopped
- 2 tablespoons olive oil
- 1 avocado, peeled, pitted, and roughly cubed
- 2 spring onions, chopped
- ¼ cup pine nuts, toasted
- 1 tablespoon balsamic vinegar
- Salt and black pepper to the taste

Directions:

1. Heat-up a pan with the oil over medium heat, add the spring onions, pine nuts, chard, stir and sauté for 5 minutes.
2. Add the vinegar and the other ingredients, toss, cook over medium heat for 10 minutes more, divide into bowls, and serve for lunch.

Nutrition: Calories 120 Fat 2g Carbs 4g Protein 8g

13. Grapes, Avocado and Spinach Salad

Preparation time: 10 minutes

Cooking time: 0 minutes

Servings: 4

Ingredients:

- 1 cup green grapes, halved
- 2 cups baby spinach
- 1 avocado, pitted, peeled, and cubed
- Salt and black pepper to the taste
- 2 tablespoons olive oil
- 1 tablespoon thyme, chopped
- 1 tablespoon rosemary, chopped
- 1 tablespoon lime juice
- 1 garlic clove, minced

Directions:

1. In a salad bowl, combine the grapes with the spinach and the other ingredients, toss, and serve for lunch.

Nutrition: Calories 190 Fat 17.1g Carbs 10.9g Protein 1.7g

14. <u>Zoodle Pesto Salad</u>

Preparation time: 15 minutes

Cooking time: 0 minutes

Servings: 2

Ingredients:

- 2 medium zucchinis (spiralized into zoodles or sliced lengthwise very thinly)
- ¼ cup extra virgin olive oil
- 1 ½ cups fresh baby spinach leaves
- ¼ cup walnuts (crushed)
- 1 tsp. garlic powder
- Sea salt and ground black pepper to taste
- ¼ cup capers (chopped)
- Optional: ½ cup of vegan cheese

Directions:

1. Combine all the ingredients except the zoodles, capers, and optional vegan cheese in a food processor or blender. Pulse for 1-2 minutes into a smooth pesto.

2. If desired, cook zoodles or zucchini slices for up to 4 minutes in a large skillet, boiling water, and a pinch of olive oil over medium heat. Alternatively, the zoodles or zucchini slices can be used raw.

3. Melt the optional vegan cheese on a plate in the microwave for about 40 seconds until it is melted and spreadable.

4. Serve the raw or cooked zoodles with the pesto, garnished with the chopped capers. Top the dish with the optional molten vegan cheese and add more salt and pepper to taste. Serve and enjoy!

Nutrition: Calories: 389 Carbs: 6.5 g. Fat: 37 g. Protein: 5.9 g.

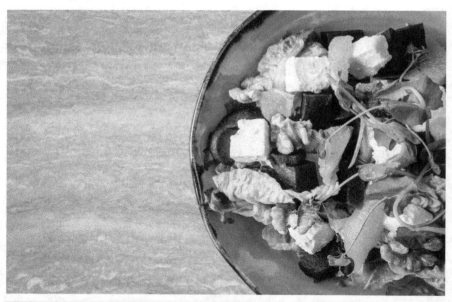

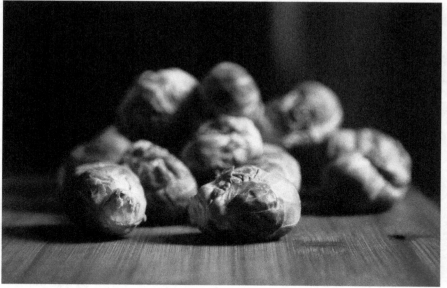

DINNER

15. <u>Zucchini Pasta</u>

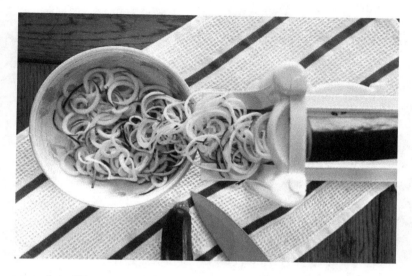

Preparation Time: 10 minutes

Cooking Time: 5 minutes

Servings: 2

Ingredients:

- 4 zucchinis, large and spiralized
- ¼ tsp. salt
- 2 avocados, chopped
- 2 tbsp. grapeseed oil
- 1 cup cherry tomatoes
- ¼ cup basil, fresh

Directions:

1. Warm-up the oil in a skillet, cook the zoodles for 5 minutes and then transfer to a large bowl. Stir in the cherry tomatoes, avocado, salt, and basil. Mix and serve.

Nutrition: Calories: 610 Fat: 53.7g Carb: 34g Protein: 9.4g

16. Egg Foo Yung

Preparation Time: 10 minutes

Cooking Time: 15 minutes

Servings: 6

Ingredients:

- Grapeseed oil as needed
- 1 cup spring water
- 1/8 tsp. ginger powder
- ½ tsp. cayenne powder
- 1 tsp. oregano
- 1 tsp. sea salt
- 1 tsp. onion powder
- 1 tsp. basil
- ¾ cup garbanzo bean flour
- ½ cup red and white onion, chopped
- ½ cup green onions, chopped
- ½ cup red and green peppers, chopped
- 1 cup butternut squash, chopped
- 2 cups mushrooms, sliced
- 3 cups prepared spaghetti squash

Directions:

1. In a bowl, whisk the garbanzo flour, seasonings, and spring water. Then add the veggies and prepared spaghetti squash. Combine to mix.
2. Coat a skillet with grapeseed oil and add ½ cup of the mixture to the pan. Pat down the dough into patties and cook 3 to 4 minutes on each side. Serve.

Nutrition: Calories: 139 Fat: 2.1g Carb: 24.7g Protein: 6.6g

17. Lentil & Chickpeas Salad

Preparation time: 15 minutes

Cooking time: 35 minutes

Servings: 6

Ingredients:

- Lentils:
- 4 cups water
- 2 cups dried green lentils, rinsed
- 2 large garlic cloves, halved lengthwise
- 2 tablespoons olive oil
- Dressing:
- 1 garlic clove, minced
- ¼ cup fresh lemon juice
- 2 tablespoons olive oil
- 1 teaspoon maple syrup
- 1 teaspoon Dijon mustard
- Salt and ground black pepper, to taste
- Salad:
- 1½ (15-ounce) cans chickpeas, rinsed and drained
- 2 large avocados, peeled, pitted, and chopped
- 2 cups radishes, trimmed and sliced
- ¼ cup fresh mint leaves, chopped

Directions:

1. For lentil, add all ingredients in a medium pot over medium-high heat and bring to a boil.

2. Then, adjust the heat to low and simmer for about 25–35 minutes or until the lentils are cooked through and tender. Drain the lentils and discard the garlic cloves.

3. For dressing, add all ingredients in a small bowl and beat until well combined. In a large serving bowl, add lentils, chickpeas, radishes, avocados, and mint, and mix. Add dressing and toss to coat well. Serve immediately.

Nutrition: Calories 561 Fat 22.2 g Carbs 66.4 g Protein 24.9 g

18. Red Beans & Corn Salad

Preparation time: 15 minutes

Cooking time: 0 minutes

Servings: 6

Ingredients:

- Dressing:
- 5 tablespoons olive oil
- 4 tablespoons fresh lime juice
- 1 tablespoon apple cider vinegar
- 3 tablespoons agave nectar
- Salt and ground black pepper, to taste
- Salad:
- 3 (15-ounce) cans red kidney beans, drained and rinsed
- 1 (15¼-ounce) can corn, drained and rinsed
- 2 cups cherry tomatoes, halved
- 1¼ cups onion, sliced
- 1/3 cup fresh cilantro, minced
- 8 cups lettuce, torn

Directions:

1. For dressing, add all ingredients in a small bowl and beat until well combined.

2. In a large serving bowl, add beans, corn, cilantro, and lettuce, and mix. Add dressing and toss to coat well. Serve immediately.

Nutrition: Calories 396 Fat 12.6 g Carbs 59.9 g Protein 17.1 g

19. **Quinoa with Veggies**

Preparation time: 15 minutes

Cooking time: 25 minutes

Servings: 3

Ingredients:

- Roasted Mushrooms:
- 2 cups small fresh Baby Bella mushrooms
- 1 tablespoon olive oil
- Salt, to taste
- Quinoa:
- 2 cups water
- 1 cup quinoa, rinsed
- 2 tablespoons fresh parsley, chopped
- 1 garlic clove, minced
- 1 tablespoon olive oil
- 2 teaspoons fresh lemon juice
- Salt and ground black pepper, to taste
- Bowl:
- 1 cup broccoli florets
- 1 cup fresh baby spinach leaves
- 2 scallions (green part), chopped
- 2 tablespoons coconut flakes
- 2 tablespoons olive oil

Directions:

1. Preheat the oven to 425°F. Prepare a large rimmed baking sheet lined using baking paper. In a bowl, add the mushrooms, oil, and salt, and toss to coat well.

2. Arrange the mushroom onto the prepared baking sheet in a single layer. Roast for about 15–18 minutes, tossing once halfway through.

3. For quinoa, add the water and quinoa in a pan over medium-high heat and bring to a boil. Adjust the heat to low and simmer, covered for about 15–20 minutes or until all the liquid is absorbed.

4. Remove from the heat and set the pan aside, covered for about 5 minutes. Uncover the pan and with a fork, the quinoa.

5. Stir in the parsley, garlic, oil, lemon juice, salt, and black pepper and set aside to cool completely.

6. For broccoli, arrange a steamer basket in a pan with the water and boil. Place the broccoli florets in steamer basket and steam, covered for about 5–6 minutes.

7. Drain the broccoli florets and set aside to cool. Divide the quinoa, mushrooms, broccoli, spinach, scallion, and coconut into serving bowls and drizzle with oil.

8. Serve immediately.

Nutrition: Calories 428 Fat 25.1 g Carbs 42.6 g Protein 12 g

20. Black Beans Stew

Preparation time: 15 minutes

Cooking time: 30 minutes

Servings: 4

Ingredients:

- 1 tablespoon olive oil
- 2 small onions, chopped
- 5 garlic cloves, chopped finely
- 1 teaspoon of dried oregano
- 1 teaspoon ground cumin
- ½ teaspoon ground ginger
- Salt and ground black pepper, to taste
- 1 (14-ounce) can diced tomatoes
- 2 (13½-ounce) cans black beans, rinsed and drained
- ½ cup vegetable broth

Directions:

1. Heat the olive oil in a pan over medium heat and cook the onion for about 5–7 minutes, stirring frequently. Add garlic, oregano, spices, salt, and black pepper and cook for about 1 minute.

2. Add the tomatoes and cook for about 1–2 minutes. Add in the beans and broth and bring to a boil. Now, adjust

the heat to medium-low and simmer, covered for about 15 minutes. Serve hot.

Nutrition: Calories 247 Fat 5.5 g Carbs 39.4 g Protein 13 g

21. **Mustard Beets**

Preparation Time: 10 minutes

Cooking Time: 0 minutes

Servings: 4

Ingredients:

- 1 tablespoon Dijon mustard
- 1 and ½ tablespoon olive oil
- 8 ounces beets, cooked and sliced
- 1 teaspoon garam masala
- 1 teaspoon coriander, ground
- 1 teaspoon basil, dried
- A pinch of black pepper

Directions:

1. Mix the beets with the oil, mustard and the other ingredients in a bowl, toss and serve.

Nutrition: Calories 170 Fat 5g Carbs 8g Proteins 5.5g

22. **Parsley Green Beans**

Preparation Time: 10 minutes

Cooking Time: 20 minutes

Servings: 6

Ingredients:

- 3 tablespoons olive oil
- 3 pounds green beans, halved
- A pinch of salt and black pepper
- 2 tablespoons balsamic vinegar
- 2 yellow onions, chopped
- 2 and ½ tablespoons parsley, chopped

Directions:

1. Warm-up a pan with the oil over medium heat, add the green beans and the other ingredients, toss, cook for 20 minutes, divide between plates and serve.

Nutrition: Calories 130 Fat 1g Carbs 7.4g Protein 6g

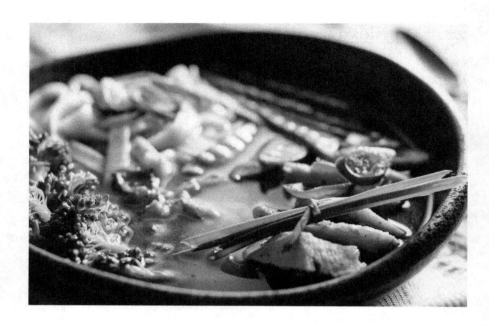

SNACKS

23. 5-Ingredient Granola Bars

Preparation time: 35 minutes

Cooking time: 0 minutes

Servings: 12

Ingredients:

- ½ cup peanut butter, almond/cashew butter/sunflower seed butter
- ¼ cup maple syrup/Simple Syrup
- ¼ cup plant-based protein powder or ground almonds
- 1½ cup rolled oats
- ¼ cup dried cranberries

Directions:

1. Stir the peanut butter and maple syrup in a large bowl until smooth. Put the protein powder, oats, plus cranberries, and mix.

2. Press the batter into an 8-inch baking dish then refrigerate within 15 minutes. Cut into 12 bars.

3. These will keep in an airtight container in the refrigerator for up to 1 week or at room temperature for about 4 days.

Nutrition: Calories: 151 Protein: 7g Fat: 6g Carbohydrates: 19g

24. **Banana–Chocolate Chip Muffins**

Preparation time: 15 minutes

Cooking time: 20-25 minutes

Servings: 12

Ingredients:

- 2 tablespoons coconut oil or vegan margarine, melted, plus more for coating the muffin tin (optional)
- 3 bananas
- ½ cup nondairy milk or plain nondairy yogurt
- ½ cup granulated sugar or packed dark brown sugar
- 2 tablespoons ground flaxseed
- 1 teaspoon vanilla extract
- 1 teaspoon apple cider vinegar
- Pinch salt
- 1 cup all-purpose flour
- 1 cup whole-wheat flour
- 1 teaspoon baking powder
- ½ teaspoon baking soda
- ½ cup vegan dark chocolate chips

Directions:

1. Preheat the oven to 400°F. Coat a muffin tin with coconut oil, line it with paper muffin cups, or use a nonstick tin.

2. In a large bowl, mash the bananas with a fork. Stir in the milk, sugar, flaxseed, coconut oil, vanilla, vinegar, and salt.

3. Add the all-purpose and whole-wheat flours, baking powder, and baking soda, stir until just combined. Fold in the chocolate chips without stirring too much.

4. Scoop the mixture into the prepared tin, about 1/3 cup for each muffin. Bake for 20 to 25 minutes, until slightly browned on top and springy to the touch.

5. Let cool for about 10 minutes. Run a dinner knife around the inside of each cup to loosen, then tilt the muffins on their sides in the muffin wells so air gets underneath. Serve.

Nutrition: Calories: 300 Protein: 7g Fat: 8g Carbohydrates: 53g

25. <u>Carrot, Pumpkin Seed & Raisin Muffins</u>

Preparation time: 15 minutes

Cooking time: 20-25 minutes

Servings: 12

Ingredients:

- 2 tablespoons coconut oil or vegan margarine, softened, plus more for preparing the muffin tin (optional)
- 1 cup nondairy milk
- 2 tablespoons ground flaxseed
- 2 teaspoons apple cider vinegar
- ½ cup sugar
- 1 tablespoon pumpkin pie spice or ground cinnamon
- Pinch salt
- 2 cups all-purpose flour
- 1 teaspoon baking powder
- ½ teaspoon baking soda
- 2 cups peeled and grated carrot
- ½ cup raisins
- ½ cup unsalted raw pumpkin seeds

Directions:

1. Preheat the oven to 400°F. Coat a muffin tin with coconut oil, line it with paper muffin cups, or use a nonstick tin.
2. In a large bowl, stir together the milk, flaxseed, coconut oil, vinegar, sugar, pumpkin pie spice, and salt.
3. Add the flour, baking powder, and baking soda, stir until just combined. Fold in the carrot, raisins, and pumpkin seeds, mixing until just combined.
4. Scoop the mixture into the prepared tin, about 1/3 cup for each muffin. Bake for 20 to 25 minutes, until slightly browned on top and springy to the touch.
5. Let cool for about 10 minutes. Run a dinner knife around the inside of each cup to loosen, then tilt the muffins on their sides in the muffin wells so air gets underneath. Serve.

Nutrition: Calories: 270 Protein: 8g Fat: 8g Carbohydrates: 45g

26.   **Spiced and Herbs Nuts**

Preparation Time: 10 Minutes

Cooking Time: 12 Minutes

Servings: 12

Ingredients:

- 1½ cups whole almonds
- 1½ cups pistachios
- 1 cup pecan halves
- 1 cup walnut halves
- 1 cup cashews
- 1/3 cup extra-virgin olive oil
- 2 tablespoons fresh rosemary, chopped
- 2 tablespoons fresh thyme, chopped
- 2 tablespoons fresh oregano, chopped
- 1 tablespoon smoked paprika
- 1 teaspoon cayenne pepper
- 2 teaspoons garlic powder
- Salt, to taste

Directions:

1. Warm your oven to 350°F and line a large baking sheet with parchment paper. In a bowl, place all ingredients and toss to coat well.

2. Transfer the nut mixture onto the prepared baking sheet and spread in a single layer. Roast for about 10–12 minutes, flipping after every 5 minutes.

3. Remove from the oven and set the baking sheet aside to cool completely before serving.

Nutrition: Calories: 369 Fat: 34g Carbohydrates: 12g Protein: 10g

27. **Hearts of Palm & Cheese Dip**

Preparation time: 15 minutes

Cooking time: 25 minutes

Servings: 9

Ingredients:

- ¼ cup mayonnaise
- ¼ cup Parmesan cheese, for topping
- ½ cup Parmesan cheese, shredded
- 1 (14-ounce) can hearts of palm, drained
- 2 large organic eggs, separate 1 of the eggs
- 2 tablespoons Italian seasoning
- 3 stalks green onions, chopped

Directions:

1. Oiled a small baking dish with cooking spray and preheat oven to 350F. In food processor, add hearts of palm, mayo, Parmesan cheese, seasoning, and green onions. Process until chopped thoroughly.
2. Add 1 egg yolk and one whole egg. Pulse four times. Pour mixture into prepared dish. Pop in the oven and bake within 20 minutes.

3. Remove from oven and mix. Top with cheese. Return to oven and broil until tops are golden brown, around 2 to 3 minutes.

Nutrition: Calories: 74 Protein: 4.9g Carbs: 4.2g Fat: 9.2g

VEGETABLES

28. Lemon Broccoli Rabe

Preparation Time: 10 minutes

Cooking Time: 10 minutes

Serving: 4

Ingredient:

- 8 cups water
- Sea salt
- 2 bunches broccoli rabe, chopped
- 3 tablespoons olive oil
- 3 garlic cloves, minced
- Pinch of cayenne pepper
- Zest of 1 lemon

Direction

1. Boil 8 cups of the water. Sprinkle a pinch of salt and the broccoli rabe. Cook until the broccoli rabe is slightly softened, about 2 minutes. Drain.

2. Heat olive oil over medium-high heat. Cook the garlic for 30 seconds. Stir in the broccoli rabe, cayenne, and lemon zest.

3. Season with salt and black pepper. Serve immediately.

Nutrition: 99 Calories 7g Fiber 11g Protein

29. Spicy Swiss Chard

Preparation Time: 10 minutes

Cooking Time: 10 minutes

Serving: 4

Ingredient:

- 2 tablespoons olive oil
- 1 onion, chopped
- 2 bunches Swiss chard
- 3 garlic cloves, minced
- ½ teaspoon red pepper flakes (or to taste)
- Juice of ½ lemon

Direction

1. In a big pot, cook olive oil over medium-high heat until it shimmers. Cook the onion and chard stems for 5 minutes.
2. Cook chard leaves for 1 minute. Stir in the garlic and pepper flakes. Cover and cook for 5 minutes. Stir in the lemon juice. Season with salt and serve immediately.

Nutrition: 94 Calories 5g Fiber 7g Protein

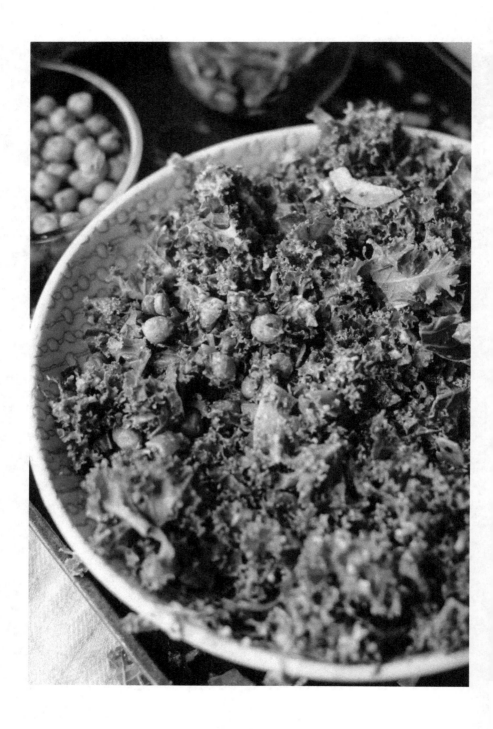

SALAD

30. **Roasted Almond Protein Salad**

Preparation Time: 30 minutes

Cooking Time: 0 minutes

Servings: 4

Ingredients:

- ½ cup dry quinoa
- ½ cup dry navy beans
- ½ cup dry chickpeas
- ½ cup raw whole almonds
- 1 tsp. extra virgin olive oil
- ½ tsp. salt
- ½ tsp. paprika
- ½ tsp. cayenne
- Dash of chili powder
- 4 cups spinach, fresh or frozen
- ¼ cup purple onion, chopped

Directions:

1. Prepare the quinoa according to the recipe. Store in the fridge for now.

2. Prepare the beans according to the method. Store in the fridge for now.

3. Toss the almonds, olive oil, salt, and spices in a large bowl, and stir until the ingredients are evenly coated.

4. Put a skillet over medium-high heat, and transfer the almond mixture to the heated skillet.

5. Roast while stirring until the almonds are browned, around 5 minutes. You may hear the ingredients pop and crackle in the pan as they warm up. Stir frequently to prevent burning.

6. Turn off the heat and toss the cooked and chilled quinoa and beans, onions, spinach, or mixed greens in the skillet. Stir well before transferring the roasted almond salad to a bowl.

7. Enjoy the salad with a dressing of choice, or, store for later!

Nutrition: Calories 347 Total Fat 10.5g Saturated Fat 1g Cholesterol 0mg Sodium 324mg Total Carbohydrate 49.2g Dietary Fiber 14.7g Total Sugars 4.7g Protein 17.2g Vitamin D 0mcg Calcium 139mg Iron 5mg Potassium 924mg

GRAINS

31. Black-Eyed Pea, Beet, and Carrot Stew

Preparation Time: 15 minutes

Cooking Time: 40 minutes

Servings: 2

Ingredients:

- ½ cup black-eyed peas, soaked in water overnight
- 3 cups water
- 1 large beet, peeled and cut into ½-inch pieces (about ¾ cup)
- 1 large carrot, peeled and cut into ½-inch pieces (about ¾ cup)
- ¼ teaspoon turmeric
- ¼ teaspoon toasted and ground cumin seeds
- 1/8 teaspoon asafetida
- ¼ cup finely chopped parsley
- ¼ teaspoon cayenne pepper
- ¼ teaspoon salt (optional)
- ½ teaspoon fresh lime juice

Directions:

1. Pour the black-eyed peas and water in a pot, then cook over medium heat for 25 minutes.
2. Add the beet and carrot to the pot and cook for 10 more minutes. Add more water if necessary.
3. Add the turmeric, cumin, asafetida, parsley, and cayenne pepper to the pot and cook for an additional 6 minutes or until the vegetables are soft. Stir the mixture periodically. Sprinkle with salt, if desired.
4. Drizzle the lime juice on top before serving in a large bowl.

Nutrition: calories: 84 | fat: 0.7g | carbs: 16.6g | protein: 4.1g | fiber: 4.5g

32. **Koshari**

Preparation Time: 15 minutes

Cooking Time: 2 hours 10 minutes

Servings: 6

Ingredients:

- 1 cup green lentils, rinsed
- 3 cups water
- Salt, to taste (optional)
- 1 large onion, peeled and minced
- 2 tablespoons low-sodium vegetable broth
- 4 cloves garlic, peeled and minced
- ½ teaspoon ground allspice
- 1 teaspoon ground coriander
- 1 teaspoon ground cumin
- 2 tablespoons tomato paste
- ½ teaspoon crushed red pepper flakes
- 3 large tomatoes, diced
- 1 cup cooked medium-grain brown rice
- 1 cup whole-grain elbow macaroni, cooked, drained, and kept warm
- 1 tablespoon brown rice vinegar

Directions:

1. Put the lentils and water in a saucepan, and sprinkle with salt, if desired. Bring to a boil over high heat. Reduce the heat to medium, then put the pan lid on and cook for 45 minutes or until the water is mostly absorbed. Pour the cooked lentils in the bowl and set aside.

2. Add the onion to a nonstick skillet, then sauté over medium heat for 15 minutes or caramelized.

3. Add vegetable broth and garlic to the skillet and sauté for 3 minutes or until fragrant.

4. Add the allspice, coriander, cumin, tomato paste, and red pepper flakes to the skillet and sauté for an additional 3 minutes until aromatic.

5. Add the tomatoes to the skillet and sauté for 15 minutes or until the tomatoes are wilted. Sprinkle with salt, if desired.

6. Arrange the cooked brown rice on the bottom of a large platter, then top the rice with macaroni, and then spread the lentils over.

7. Pour the tomato mixture and brown rice vinegar over before serving.

Nutrition: calories: 201 fat: 1.6g carbs: 41.8g protein: 6.5g fiber: 3.

LEGUMES

33. <u>Old-Fashioned Chili</u>

Preparation Time: 10 minutes

Cooking Time: 10 minutes

Servings: 4

Ingredients:

- 3/4-pound red kidney beans, soaked overnight
- 2 tablespoons olive oil
- 1 onion, chopped
- 2 bell peppers, chopped
- 1 red chili pepper, chopped
- 2 ribs celery, chopped
- 2 cloves garlic, minced
- 2 bay leaves
- 1 teaspoon ground cumin
- 1 teaspoon thyme, chopped
- 1 teaspoon black peppercorns
- 20 ounces' tomatoes, crushed
- 2 cups vegetable broth
- 1 teaspoon smoked paprika
- Sea salt, to taste

- 2 tablespoons fresh cilantro, chopped
- 1 avocado, pitted, peeled and sliced

Directions:

1. Cover the soaked beans with a fresh change of cold water and bring to a boil. Let it boil for about 10 minutes. Turn the heat to a simmer and continue to cook for 50 to 55 minutes or until tender.

2. In a heavy-bottomed pot, heat the olive oil over medium heat. Once hot, sauté the onion, bell pepper and celery.

3. Sauté the garlic, bay leaves, ground cumin, thyme and black peppercorns for about 1 minute or so.

4. Add in the diced tomatoes, vegetable broth, paprika, salt and cooked beans. Let it simmer, stirring periodically, for 25 to 30 minutes or until cooked through.

5. Serve garnished with fresh cilantro and avocado. Bon appétit!

Nutrition: Calories: 514; Fat: 16.4g; Carbs: 72g; Protein: 25.8g

34. Easy Red Lentil Salad

Preparation Time: 10 minutes

Cooking Time: 10 minutes

Servings: 4

Ingredients:

- 1/2 cup red lentils, soaked overnight and drained
- 1 ½ cups water
- 1 sprig rosemary
- 1 bay leaf
- 1 cup grape tomatoes, halved
- 1 cucumber, thinly sliced
- 1 bell pepper, thinly sliced
- 1 clove garlic, minced
- 1 onion, thinly sliced
- 2 tablespoons fresh lime juice
- 4 tablespoons olive oil
- Sea salt and ground black pepper, to taste

Directions

1. Add the red lentils, water, rosemary and bay leaf to a saucepan and bring to a boil over high heat. Then, turn the heat to a simmer and continue to cook for 20 minutes or until tender.

2. Place the lentils in a salad bowl and let them cool completely.
3. Add in the remaining ingredients and toss to combine well. Serve at room temperature or well-chilled.
4. Bon appétit!

Nutrition: Calories: 295; Fat: 18.8g; Carbs: 25.2g; Protein: 8.5g

BREAD & PIZZA

35. Keto Hamburger Buns

Preparation time: 5 minutes

Cooking time: 15 minutes

Servings: 5

Ingredients:

- 1 1/4 cup almond flour
- 1 1/2 cup mozzarella cheese, part skim grated
- 2 oz cream cheese
- 1 egg, large
- 2 tablespoons oat Fiber 500/ Protein powder
- 1 tablespoon baking powder
- 1 Metal plate or a pan which you care less about

Directions:

1. Using a microwave safe bowl, put the cream cheese and mozzarella cheese. Microwave the cheese for I minutes.

2. Remove the bowl, stir and microwave again for 40 seconds to another minute.

3. Scrape out the cheese and place it together with the egg into a food processor. Stop when it's smooth.

4. Add your dry **Ingredients,** processing it till dough is formed. (It is normally very sticky) Let the dough cool.

5. Preheat your oven to 400-degree F, placing the rack in the middle. Line your baking sheet with parchment paper and place the cheap metal plate or pan at the bottom of the oven.

6. Once the oven is ready, separate the dough into 5 equal portions. Apply oil on your hands (not too much) and roll the portions into balls.

7. Place them on the parchment paper, flattening them a bit while creating a domed shape.

8. Put 5 or 6 ice cubes on the metal pan and place the buns inside the oven. The steam from the cubes will make the buns rise.

9. Bake them for about fifteen minutes. They should be done once they brown on the outside. If not, give them more minutes in the oven.

Nutrition: Calories 294 Carbohydrates 7 g Fats 25 g Protein 14 g

36. **Paleo, Keto Buns**

Preparation time: 10 minutes

Cooking time: 45 minutes

Servings: 10

Ingredients:

- 1 1/2 cup almond meal
- 1/2 cup coconut flour
- 1/2 cup flax meal
- 2/3 cup psyllium husks
- 6 egg whites, large
- 2 eggs, large
- 5 tablespoons sesame seeds
- 2 teaspoons garlic powder
- 2 teaspoons cream of tartar/ apple cider vinegar
- 2 teaspoon onion powder
- 1 teaspoon baking soda
- 1 teaspoon sea salt/ pink Himalayan
- 2 tablespoons Erythritol
- 480 ml boiling water

Directions:

1. Preheat your oven to 350-degree F
2. Mix all your dryingredients in a mixing bowl.

3. Add your egg whites and eggs. Use a hand mixer to process it till your dough becomes thick.
4. Add the boiling water and process until it combines.
5. Line your baking sheet with parchment paper.
6. Use a spoon to make the buns and create a dome shape.
7. Sprinkle the sesame seeds on the buns. Press the seeds into the buns to prevent them from falling out.
8. Bake for 45 minutes.

Nutrition: Calories 208 Carbohydrates 9 g Fats 12 g Protein 6 g

SOUP AND STEW

37. Basic Recipe for Vegetable Broth

Preparation Time: 10 Minutes

Cooking Time: 60 Minutes

Servings: Makes 2 Quarts

Ingredients:

- 8 cups Water
- 1 Onion, chopped
- 4 Garlic cloves, crushed
- 2 Celery Stalks, chopped
- Pinch of Salt
- 1 Carrot, chopped
- Dash of Pepper
- 1 Potato, medium & chopped
- 1 tbsp. Soy Sauce
- 3 Bay Leaves

Directions:

1. To make the vegetable broth, you need to place all of the ingredients in a deep saucepan.
2. Heat the pan over a medium-high heat. Bring the vegetable mixture to a boil.

3. Once it starts boiling, lower the heat to medium-low and allow it to simmer for at least an hour or so. Cover it with a lid.

4. When the time is up, pass it through a filter and strain the vegetables, garlic, and bay leaves.

5. Allow the stock to cool completely and store in an air-tight container.

Nutrition: Calories: 44 kcal Fat: 0.6g Carbs: 9.7g Protein: 0.9g

38.   Cucumber Dill Gazpacho

Preparation Time: 10 Minutes

Cooking Time: 2 hours

Serving Size: 4

Ingredients:

- 4 large cucumbers, peeled, deseeded, and chopped
- 1/8 tsp salt
- 1 tsp chopped fresh dill + more for garnishing
- 2 tbsp freshly squeezed lemon juice
- 1 ½ cups green grape, seeds removed
- 3 tbsp extra virgin olive oil
- 1 garlic clove, minced

Directions:

1. Add all the ingredients to a food processor and blend until smooth.
2. Pour the soup into serving bowls and chill for 1 to 2 hours.
3. Garnish with dill and serve chilled.

Nutrition: Calories: 236 kcal Fat: 1.8g Carbs: 48.3g Protein: 7g

SAUCES, DRESSINGS & DIP

39. Chocolate Coconut Butter

Preparation time: 10 minutes

Cooking time: 20 minutes

Servings: 20

Ingredients:

- 1/2 lb. unsweetened shredded coconut
- 3 tablespoon cocoa butter
- 1/8 teaspoon salt

Directions:

1. Preheat your oven to 350 degrees F.
2. Place shredded coconut on a greased baking sheet. Spread out into a thin, even layer.
3. Bake for up to 15 minutes or until the coconut flakes are golden brown. Stir the coconut shreds every 3 minutes and watch them closely because they burn very easily and quickly.
4. Allow the coconut flakes to cool for 15 minutes.
5. Add coconut flakes to a food processor and blend until smooth and creamy yet runny in consistency.

6. Adding cocoa butter and salt and blend to incorporate well.

7. Pour into an airtight jar and seal lid. The consistency will thicken up as the butter cools. The oil may separate and float to the top of the container as the butter cools.

8. Simply reheat a portion in the microwave just before using. Can be stored for up to a whole year at room temperature!

Nutrition: Total fat: 17.4g Cholesterol: 0mg Sodium: 17mg Total carbohydrates: 0.9g Dietary fiber: 0.6g Protein: 0.3g

40. **Orange Dill Butter**

Preparation time: 10 minutes

Cooking time: 15 minutes

Servings: 12

Ingredients:

- 1/2 cup vegan butter

- 2 tablespoons fresh dill, finely chopped

- 2 tablespoons orange zest

- 1 teaspoon salt

Directions:

1. Add 4 cups of water to a small pot and bring to a boil over high heat. Reduce heat to low and allow water to simmer.
2. Add vegan butter to a glass Mason jar and screw on lid loosely.
3. Place Mason jar in the boiling water. Ensure that the jar does not get submerged or over turn.
4. Allow the butter to melt and add remaining Ingredients:
5. Remove the Mason jar from the pot and allow to cool until the mixture becomes partially solidified.

6. Can be used alongside your favorite veggies to infuse them with flavor and fat. Can be stored in the refrigerator for up to 2 weeks.

Nutrition: Total fat: 1.5g Cholesterol: 0mg Sodium: 199mg Total carbohydrates: 1g Dietary fiber: 0.3g Protein: 0.1g

APPETIZER

41. <u>Salt and Vinegar Chips</u>

Preparation Time: 12 hours and 10 minutes

Cooking Time: 10 minutes

Servings: 8

Ingredients:

- 1 zucchini
- 2 teaspoons of olive oil, extra virgin
- 2 tablespoons apple cider vinegar
- Himalayan salt to preference

Directions:

1. Preheat oven to 110°F. Use a knife to slice the zucchini very thin. Turn the setting to 1/8. Add the zucchini to a bowl and toss in all other ingredients.
2. Pour the zucchini onto Teflon-lined sheets. Bake and dehydrate for 12 hours until crispy.

Nutrition: Calories 13 Fat 1 g Protein 0.5 g Carbs 0 g

42. <u>Black Bean Dip</u>

Preparation Time: 15 minutes

Cooking Time: 5 minutes

Servings: 6

Ingredients:

- 15 ounces (1 can) black beans, drained and rinsed
- 2 tablespoons red onion, roughly chopped
- 1 small tomato, chopped
- 2 teaspoons garlic, minced
- ½ teaspoon cumin
- ½ lime, juiced
- Himalayan salt to preference

Directions:

1. Add all ingredients to a food processor and pulse until combined. Serve hot or warm. This recipe also makes a great dressing for salads.

Nutrition: Calories 70 Fat 0.5 g Protein 5 g Carbs 13 g

SMOOTHIES AND JUICES

43. Berry Lemonade Tea

Preparation Time: 5 minutes

Cooking Time: 12 minutes

Servings: 4

Ingredients:

- 3 tea bags
- 2 cups of natural lemonade
- 1 cup of frozen mixed berries
- 2 cups of water
- 1 lemon, sliced

Directions:

1. Put everything in the Instant Pot and cover. Cook on High for 12 minutes. Open, strain, and serve.

Nutrition: Calories 21; Carbs 8g; Fat 0.2g; Protein 0.4g

44. **Swedish Glögg**

Preparation Time: 5 minutes

Cooking Time: 15 minutes

Servings: 1

Ingredients:

- ½ cup of orange juice
- ½ cup of water
- 1 piece of ginger cut into ½ pieces
- 1 whole clove
- 1 opened cardamom pods
- 2 tbsps. orange zest
- 1 cinnamon stick
- 1 whole allspice
- 1 vanilla bean

Directions:

1. Add everything in the pot. Cover and cook on High for 15 minutes. Open and serve.

Nutrition: Calories 194; Carbs 41g; Fat 3g; Protein 1.7g

DESSERTS

45. Jasmine Rice Pudding with Dried Apricots

Preparation time: 15 minutes

Cooking time: 0 minutes

Servings: 4

Ingredients:

- 1 cup jasmine rice, rinsed
- 1 cup water
- 1 cup almond milk
- 1/2 cup brown sugar
- A pinch of salt
- A pinch of grated nutmeg
- 1/2 cup dried apricots, chopped
- 1/4 teaspoon cinnamon powder
- 1 teaspoon vanilla extract

Directions:

1. Put the rice plus water to a saucepan. Cover your saucepan then boil the water. Adjust the heat to low; simmer for another 10 minutes until all the water is absorbed.

2. Then, add in the remaining ingredients and stir to combine. Let it simmer for 10 minutes more or until the pudding has thickened. Bon appétit!

Nutrition: Calories: 300 Fat: 2.2g Carbs: 63.6g Protein: 5.6g

46. **Everyday Energy Bars**

Preparation time: 15 minutes

Cooking time: 33 minutes

Servings: 16

Ingredients:

- 1 cup vegan butter
- 1 cup brown sugar
- 2 tablespoons agave syrup
- 2 cups old-fashioned oats
- 1/2 cup almonds, slivered
- 1/2 cup walnuts, chopped
- 1/2 cup dried currants
- 1/2 cup pepitas

Directions:

1. Warm your oven to 320 degrees F. Line a baking pan with parchment paper or Silpat mat. Thoroughly combine all the ingredients until everything is well incorporated.

2. Spread the mixture onto the prepared baking pan using a wide spatula. Bake for about 33 minutes or until golden brown.

3. Slice into bars using a sharp knife and enjoy!

Nutrition: Calories: 285 Fat: 17.1g Carbs: 30g Protein: 5.1g

47. <u>Chocolate Hazelnut Fudge</u>

Preparation time: 1 hour & 15 minutes

Cooking time: 0 minutes

Servings: 20

Ingredients:

- 1 cup cashew butter
- 1 cup fresh dates, pitted
- 1/4 cup cocoa powder
- 1/4 teaspoon ground cloves
- 1 teaspoon matcha powder
- 1 teaspoon vanilla extract
- 1/2 cup hazelnuts, coarsely chopped

Directions:

1. Process all ingredients in your blender until uniform and smooth.
2. Scrape the batter into a parchment-lined baking sheet.
3. Place it in your freezer for at least 1 hour to set.
4. Cut into squares and serve.

5. Bon appétit!

Nutrition: Calories: 127 Fat: 9g Carbs: 10.7g Protein: 2.4g

48. No-Bake Pumpkin Pie

Preparation Time: 10 minutes

Cooking Time: 0 minutes

Servings: 8

Ingredients:

- 1 cup pumpkin puree
- 2 tsp pumpkin pie spice
- oz. vanilla pudding
- 8-ounce cool whip
- ¼ cup milk
- 1 graham cracker crust
- Whipped cream for garnish

Directions:

1. Take a bowl pour pumpkin puree in it, add pudding mix, pumpkin pie spice and milk. Mix the Ingredients well until they turn smooth.
2. Now fold it into cool whip carefully. Take a graham cracker in a pie pan and spread the pumpkin puree on the pie and spread well.

3. Chill it well before serving, and serve with whipped cream topping.

Nutrition: Calories: 323 Carbs: 42g Fat: 15g Protein: 6g

49. <u>Vegan Vanilla Almond Cookies</u>

Preparation Time: 15 minutes

Cooking Time: 45 minutes

Servings: 10

Ingredients:

- 2 cups all-purpose flour
- 1 cup almond meal
- ½ tsp. salt
- 1 cup powdered sugar
- 1 cup vegan butter
- ½ tsp. almond extract
- 2 tsp. vanilla
- 20 almonds

Directions:

1. Warm your oven to 350 degrees Fahrenheit. Mix your dry fixings in a large bowl. Put the wet fixings, and stir well to create a dough. Don't add the almonds.
2. Next, roll your dough into a log with a two-inch diameter, and slice the cookie roll into flat cookies— like you would slice a cucumber.
3. Put the cookies on your baking sheet, and press the almonds into the cookies.

4. Bake the cookies within 20 minutes in the preheated oven, and enjoy.

Nutrition: Calories: 180 Carbs: 13g Fat: 14g Protein: 4g

50. Mocha Fudge

Preparation time: 1 hour & 15 minutes

Cooking time: 0 minutes

Servings: 20

Ingredients:

- 1 cup cookies, crushed
- 1/2 cup almond butter
- 1/4 cup agave nectar
- 6 ounces dark chocolate, broken into chunks
- 1 teaspoon instant coffee
- A pinch of grated nutmeg
- A pinch of salt

Directions:

1. Prepare a large baking sheet lined using parchment paper. Melt the chocolate in your microwave and add in the remaining ingredients; stir to combine well.
2. Scrape the batter into a parchment-lined baking sheet. Place it in your freezer for at least 1 hour to set. Cut into squares and serve.

3. Bon appétit!

Nutrition: Calories: 105 Fat: 5.6g Carbs: 12.9g Protein: 1.1g

CPSIA information can be obtained
at www.ICGtesting.com
Printed in the USA
LVHW082011190421
684916LV00010B/491

9 781801 832892